Understanding Adult ADHD

From Signs and Symptoms to Causes and Diagnosis

Christine Weil

Table of Contents

Introduction

I want to thank you and congratulate you for purchasing, *"Natural Health & Natural Cures Series - Understanding Adult ADHD."*

This book contains valuable information that will help you understand adult ADHD.

If you are reading this guide, then chances are either you or someone close to you is experiencing symptoms of adult ADHD or has recently been diagnosed with adult ADHD. The information provided here will explain what adult ADHD is, outline the common symptoms those with the condition experience, and explain the process used to diagnose the disorder. You will want to keep this guide handy as a quick reference guide as you learn more about managing and treating adult ADHD.

Thank you again for purchasing this book.

I hope you enjoy it!

Christine Weil

What is Adult ADHD?

ADHD in general may be one of the most researched and yet still most misunderstood mental health conditions afflicting members of our society. Despite being the most researched mental health condition in children, there is still much we don't know about ADHD, especially when it comes to how it affects adults. In order to understand this condition and make the best choices about getting help and support for the symptoms and problems it causes, we need to have a basic understanding of what it is and what it isn't. So, here is what we do know, based on the currently available research.

What We Know About ADHD

1. ADHD is a brain-based disorder.

ADHD or the collection of symptoms we call ADHD results from neurological differences in the brain. We know that children with ADHD exhibit different levels of specific neurotransmitters than children without ADHD. We can only assume that the same is true for adults with the condition since there has been very little research into ADHD in adults. We also know that the reward system of the brain, which produces and utilizes dopamine, seems to work differently in ADHD brains than it does in brains without ADHD.

2. ADHD is a life-long condition.

For years, the generally accepted belief was that only adolescents had ADHD and that as they grew into adulthood they "outgrew" it. It is only within the last decade that the mental health community has truly embraced the idea that

ADHD persists into adulthood. The reason we used to believe that people outgrew the disorder is because ADHD looks different in adults than it does in children. Additionally, a percentage of people with ADHD will adopt coping mechanisms, create environments, or build lives as adults that minimize the impact of their ADHD, effectively neutralizing the negative impact the disorder has on their lives. In these people, the childhood condition will therefore seem to have disappeared.

3. ADHD affects people differently.

One of the challenges of ADHD, in both children and adults, is that the disorder affects people differently. While most other health conditions have a group of symptoms that everyone with the condition will experience, ADHD has a group of symptoms that not everyone with the disorder will experience, either the same amount of symptoms nor to the same degree. This is one reason that the myth that ADHD doesn't actually exist persists.

4. Executive functioning is at the root of ADHD.

The term "executive function" is used to describe our brain's management system. This system is what allows us to plan, organize, prioritize, remember, focus, understand, and engage. The generally accepted list of executive functions includes:

- Inhibition
- Self-talk
- Initiation
- Foresight/Hindsight
- Flexibility
- Organization

- Working Memory
- Motivation
- Emotional regulation
- Sense of time

An ADHD brain has difficulty with one or more of these executive functions, and all the symptoms generally associated with ADHD tie back to challenges in one of these areas.

5. ADHD is a situationally-based condition.

Another reason that the "ADHD isn't real" myth continues to be perpetuated is that people with ADHD can excel in one area and fail miserably in others, even in areas that seem similar to outsiders. For this reason, ADHD is considered to be a situationally-based condition. This is why someone with ADHD can spending five hours reading a novel without once looking up from the book even though they cannot spend more than 10 minutes reading something for work. Situationally-based is not the same as erratic. Generally speaking, the situations where someone with ADHD excels or fails will be the same, if you understand the underlying executive function that drives that success or that failure.

6. ADHD creates strengths and weaknesses.

While most of the discussion about ADHD focuses on the challenges and obstacles it causes, it can also come with gifts. People with ADHD can be brilliant and extremely successful in some areas of their lives, while also being very unsuccessful and struggling in other areas of their lives. Understanding all the ways that ADHD impacts a person's life is the key to successfully learning to manage it.

7. ADHD affects between 5-10% of the population.

The jury is still out on the actual prevalence of the condition but most experts agree that the real number lies somewhere between 5 and 10%. Most statistics use 4% as the part of the adult population with the disorder, but if you accept the idea that people do not actually "outgrow" it, the number for children and adults should be the same.

8. ADHD affects both girls and boys, both women and men.

For a long time, ADHD was believed to impact boys at a higher rate than girls. However, as the understanding of the disorder has broadened, we are beginning to see that boys are more likely to be diagnosed in childhood, which makes it seem like they are more susceptible. This is primarily because boys are more likely than girls to be hyperactive. However, as more and more women are diagnosed as adults, that trend is expected to change.

ADD vs. ADHD

One of the things that people often find confusing is the use of the terms ADD and the ADHD. While ADHD was previously used to differentiate those who had this condition with hyperactivity, the DSM-V groups all attention deficit disorder symptoms under one category. It's called attention deficit and hyperactivity disorder or ADHD, regardless of whether or not the person experiences the hyperactive side of the condition.

ADHD Subtypes

Within the ADHD diagnosis, there are three generally accepted subtypes of the disorder – primarily hyperactive-impulsive, primarily inattentive, and combined. When someone is diagnosed with ADHD, they may or may not be told which sub-type they have. While knowing which subtype may be informational, it isn't necessary in order to learn to manage the condition since it is such an individual disorder.

How Does ADHD Affect the Brain?

Although there is much research that remains to be done before we can truly say we understand how ADHD impacts the human brain, we do know that the way dopamine works in an ADHD brain is different than in a non-ADHD brain.

Dopamine is a neurotransmitter that seems to be responsible for mental stimulation and that works with the brain's reward system.   Research indicates that adults with ADHD have different levels of dopamine than their non-ADHD peers, generally less, and that their dopamine release/response system doesn't always work the way it is expected to. This can mean that an ADHD brain isn't making enough dopamine, that the dopamine being made is getting used up more quickly than it should, or that an ADHD brain simply requires a higher amount of dopamine to get the same result.

Understanding the dopamine connection is important on several levels.

First, it helps provide a basis of understanding for many of the symptoms seen in adult ADHD. For example, those with ADHD are more likely to be risk-takers and to participate in exciting and even dangerous activities. If you understand the dopamine connection, it becomes easier to see that those with ADHD are more likely to take risks because risky behavior results in the release of more dopamine. Where someone without ADHD can ride a bike down a hill with their family, someone with ADHD may need to ride their bike 60 mph downhill to get the same effect.

The dopamine connection also helps explain why stimulant medications, which are covered later, help people with ADHD. These kinds of medication provide the ADHD brain with extra dopamine or help the brain handle the dopamine it already has, more appropriately.

The dopamine connection also has a downside, however. Illegal drugs and other substances that can lead to substance abuse problems also produce a temporary increase in the dopamine levels in the brain. Initial research indicates that this may be why those with ADHD are more susceptible to suffering from substance abuse problems at some point during their life.

What are the Signs and Symptoms of Adult ADHD?

ADHD is a collection of symptoms related to executive functioning. As adults with ADHD can have any combination of these symptoms, the signs of ADHD in one person can be very different than the signs in someone else. To illustrate, here are some of the "signs" that can indicate someone may be struggling with adult ADHD.

Common Signs of Adult ADHD

- Constantly making simple errors at work despite being previously corrected
- Consistently forgetting to pay bills, file income taxes, or send permission slips into school
- Sacrificing accuracy for speed on tedious or boring tasks
- Unwillingness to check work for errors once a task is completed
- Difficulty sticking with a task until it is completed
- Jumping from one task to another
- Impulsively quitting their job more than once
- Struggling to remain engaged in long conversations
- Finding it difficult to maintain focus on even enjoyable activities for an extended timeframe
- Consistently experiencing difficulty listening to others and retaining the information imparted to them
- Consistently struggling to follow both written and verbal instructions from others
- Seeming to be tuned-out to the extent that people must touch them or say their name several times to get their attention

- Being consistently late for meetings, events, engagements, and appointments
- Being forgetful
- Frequently losing or misplacing things
- Consistently procrastinating, especially on things that are time-consuming, mental challenging, or boring
- Finding it difficult to sit in traffic or wait in line
- Being easily distracted by external stimuli
- Finding it difficult to stop doing something when it is time to switch to a different activity
- Being irritable and easy to anger
- Finding it difficult to sit still
- Frequently tapping their foot, a pencil, or performing some other repetitive physical action
- Finding it difficult to remain quiet during movies or other activities where quiet is required
- Being unable to relax, even on vacation
- Consistently interrupting others during conversations or talking over people
- Finding it difficult to wait for others who cannot maintain the frenetic pace they prefer
- Frequently saying things without thinking and being seen often as lacking tact
- Failing to live up to their potential

Symptoms Associated with Adult ADHD

Each of these signs relates back to one or more of the common symptoms seen in adults with ADHD. One of the challenges ADHD presents from both a diagnosis and treatment standpoint is that the symptoms often overlap and intertwine to create even more symptoms or to exacerbate existing symptoms. This is because of the inter-related nature of executive functioning. Our executive functions also overlap and work together, which means that when one or more of them is not working as expected, there can be a ripple effect.

Inattention

Inattention in ADHD is best described as the inability to pay close attention to details. For adults this can cause problems in every area of their lives. It can result in poor performance at work, especially if they work in a job where attention to detail is required. Inattention can also contribute to problems with working and prospective memory (mentioned later) as you cannot remember things you don't pay attention to in the first place.

People who struggle with inattention can be seen as daydreamers and are prone to making careless mistakes simply because of their lack of attention. When someone who struggles with inattention has to perform a detail-intensive task, it can be very stressful, which only exacerbates their ADHD symptoms.

Another part of inattention is the inability to sustain attention for the required amount of time. Some adults with ADHD will find it very difficult to keep their attention focused on one task or activity for an extended period of time. The inability to sustain attention contributes to other symptoms like the inability to finish things.

Poor Listening Skills

Many people with ADHD struggle to actively and effectively listen to other people. This can happen for a variety of reasons. It may be that the person has difficulty processing verbal information. It may also be that they find it challenging to keep their attention focused on what the other person is saying. Working memory can also mask itself as poor listening. If someone struggles to remember information that is provided verbally, like instructions, it can seem as though the person didn't listen initially, when the problem is really a problem with working memory.

People who struggle with listening will find it very difficult to follow verbal directions, especially if those directions are given as a list of tasks all at once. They may only be able to focus on the first two or three items. This may mean that they perform the first couple of tasks and then switch to something else without realizing that they haven't actually completed the task at hand.

Poor listening can also make it difficult to remain engaged in long conversations or presentations.

Lack of Follow-Through

While people experience different ADHD symptoms, some symptoms, like this one, are fairly common across all of those with the disorder. ADHD can make it difficult to start a task and then stick with that task until it is completed. This lack of follow-through can be caused by several different factors. Finishing a task or project requires sustained attention, which can be challenging for many adults with ADHD. Additionally, seeing something all the way through to the end often requires planning and organization, which many adults with ADHD struggle to do.

The inability to follow-through on tasks often results in broken promises, unmet expectations, and missed deadlines. It can cause significant problems across all areas of life.

Procrastination

Another hallmark of adult ADHD is procrastination. People with this disorder are prone to putting off any and all tasks, especially if those tasks are too challenging, not challenging enough, boring, tedious, uninteresting, or very complex. In order to become engaged, the ADHD brain needs a burst of dopamine. When a task is unchallenging, boring, tedious, or uninteresting, the ADHD brain may simply not have enough dopamine to engage, so the task is put off for another time.

Procrastination can also happen if a task seems too big, too complicated, or too challenging. This happens when another ADHD symptom, difficulties with sequencing, leaves the person with no idea how to start the task, so they put it off simply because they don't know where to begin.

Difficulties with Planning

Planning and planning ahead are both challenges experienced by many adults with ADHD. Planning is one of the core executive functions used by the brain to manage everyday life, and the inability to plan can have significant consequences across all areas of a person's life. Difficulties with planning can stem from several base symptoms including chunking, sequencing, and working memory. Effective planning requires the ability to look at the big picture in order to see the expected end result. That big picture must be broken down into smaller detailed actions which must be placed in the correct order. Once the implementation of that plan begins, flexibility to change that plan is required. Adults with ADHD can have difficulties at each step in this process.

Translating Between the Details and the Big Picture

Most people are either big-picture people or detail-oriented people. This is also true for those with ADHD. However, where a non-ADHD adult who prefers the big picture can generally translate that big picture into individual details, this is not always the case for those with ADHD. Some ADHD adults can only grasp the big picture or the details and struggle with translating from one to the other. Those who struggle to translate a big picture into details can have difficulty with chunking and sequencing. Those who see the details and struggle to translate that to a big picture can experience communication issues and fail to meet the expectations of others.

This also contributes to difficulties with planning, organizing, and time management.

Inability to Break Tasks Down

One of the things the brain's executive functions do is to help take big things and break them down into smaller things. This is how we can go from "I want to go on vacation" to "I need to book a flight, reserve a room, and ask for time off."

The inability to break tasks down into smaller and smaller pieces can make planning, sequencing, organizing, and other things very difficult for adults with ADHD.

Struggles with Sequencing

Another important thing handled by the brain's executive functions is the sequencing of tasks. This means being able to determine the order in which a set of tasks needs to be completed so that a specified result can be achieved. For example, in order to make cookies, the brain needs to know that combining the ingredients together has to come before placing them in the oven, so the proper sequence says mix before baking. ADHD brains can't always figure out the right order of events to get from A to B so that the end result is C.

People who have difficulties with sequencing will struggle with planning, organizing, and following-through to complete tasks. They may also struggle with procrastination as sequencing can also make it challenging to determine where to start.

Difficulty Transitioning

Transitioning difficulty is something that is easier to see and understand in children, but that can create significant challenges for adults. Transitioning is the act of going from one activity to another. For a child this might mean going from math class to art class. For an adult, it can mean going from work to home or going from doing something fun to doing something obligatory. When children with ADHD struggle with transitions, it often leads to tantrums and acting out. In the world of an adult with ADHD, tantrums often look like angry outbursts, and those who have difficulty transitioning may respond by lashing out at others.

Transitioning difficulties can also occur for adults with ADHD when they have to stop doing what they want to do or have planned to do and switch over to follow some other agenda. Resistance, anxiety, anger, and refusal are other ways that adults can respond when faced with transitioning challenges.

Distractibility

Adults with ADHD may be highly distractible. This means that even subtle things that many other people may not even notice can distract ADHD adults and take them off task. Small physical things like temperature changes, the sound of someone else's phone conversation, or the smell of someone's perfume can make focusing and concentration seem impossible. Phone calls, emails, people stopping by, or any other kind of interruption can also be distracting and pull the person's attention away from the task at hand.

In addition to being easily distracted, many adults with ADHD also struggle to manage or mitigate those distractions and disruptions effectively. For example, someone without ADHD may be able to take a phone call while working on a report, talk for 15 minutes, and go right back to working on the report without really missing a beat. Meanwhile, an adult with ADHD who takes a phone call while working on a report may get distracted by the content of the phone call and jump over to a new task after hanging up the phone, completely forgetting about the report they were working on.

While most people can filter out things like the sound of the washing machine in the other room or the voice of the person in the next cube, ADHD adults that struggle with distractibility cannot filter those things out. This means that anything distracting can break their focus and seriously impact their productivity at work and at home.

Hyperfocusing

One of the most common misunderstandings of ADHD is that it is the inability to focus on or pay attention. In truth, it is more about being unable to regulate focus and attention, which is why some adults with ADHD struggle with hyperfocus.

Hyperfocusing is the opposite of not paying attention. An ADHD adult in hyperfocus mode can work on something for hours and hours without taking a break and with little awareness of the world around them. They may be so focused that it is difficult to tear their attention away. Other people may need to speak their name several times or even touch them to get their attention at all.

Hyperfocusing can be both blessing and curse as it can lead to a time of incredible productivity, but is only beneficial when the person is hyperfocused on the right thing. Additionally, hyperfocusing often comes with a cost as it can be physically and mentally exhausting. Twelve hours spent hyperfocusing can require days of downtime in order to recover.

Physical Hyperactivity

Adults with ADHD can struggle with physical hyperactivity, but it generally looks different in adults than it does in children. Where a child may be "bouncing off the walls" at school, a hyperactive adult may find it difficult to stay seated in long meetings or find they need to doodle on a piece of paper in order to stay seated. People who struggle with physical hyperactivity have a near constant need to move, especially when engaged in something boring or uninteresting. For adults, this can manifest as fidgeting, tapping, moving, talking, or engaging in some other physical activity, often without any awareness of that activity. Adults who are hyperactive may have trouble participating in activities that are not physically active. They may feel restless and are often driven to find something more active to do all the time. They also have difficulty doing things that are generally considered to be "relaxing." Feeling obligated to "relax" in these ways can cause anxiety and stress for them.

Another way that physical hyperactivity can manifest in ADHD adults is excessive talking. Telling long, elaborate stories, dominating conversations, talking during meetings or presentations, and interrupting others are all signs that an ADHD adult is struggling with physical hyperactivity.

Mental Hyperactivity

It is more common for ADHD adults to experience hyperactivity mentally rather than physically. Mental hyperactivity can cause rapid-fire thoughts that make it difficult to think straight or communicate effectively. These thoughts can be racing so fast that the person struggles to hang on to a single thought long enough to turn it into an action. Mental hyperactivity can also make focusing and sustaining attention challenging.

This kind of hyperactivity, along with the physical kind, can also create problems with impatience. The restless, need to be moving/doing something feeling that hyperactivity creates can make waiting in line, waiting in traffic, and waiting for other people annoying. This kind of impatience may lead to more physical actions geared toward alleviating the hyperactivity being experienced. For example, someone waiting in line at the store may start shifting their weight from side to side, picking at their finger nails, or tapping their feet.

Difficulty Organizing

Many adults with ADHD struggle with organizing everything from the thoughts in their head to the clothes in their closet. Organizing is one of the executive functions and when an adult with ADHD has difficulty with organization, it can exacerbate almost every other ADHD symptom. In essence, organizing is about grouping things together in a way that makes sense to the person, and that makes them easier to retrieve/use in the future. This requires a big picture, details, hindsight, foresight, planning, breaking down tasks, sequencing, and several other skills and abilities many ADHD adults struggle with.

Forgetfulness

Many ADHD adults struggle with forgetfulness. This can range from forgetting to pay bills to forgetting where they parked their car to forgetting to pick their child up after dance class. These kinds of problems stem from issues with working memory, prospective memory, and inattention.

This kind of forgetfulness can result in frequently losing things, misplacing things, forgetting about appointments, missing birthdays and anniversaries, and many other problems. It can also cause problems in the workplace if deadlines are missed because they are forgotten or important work products are misplaced.

Impulsivity

Impulsivity is the inability to moderate one's own behavior so that the right thing is done at the right time. For adults with ADHD, impulse behavior can include which can blurting things out in meetings, talking over other people, being impatient, taking foolish risks with finances or business, engaging in risky or dangerous activities, being unfaithful in relationships, using or abusing substances, and making poorly thought out decisions.

Adults with ADHD who struggle with impulsivity may buy things they can't afford, struggle to follow a budget, and find it difficult to sustain a monogamous relationship over time.

All or Nothing Thinking

Another common symptom that ADHD adults can experience is all or nothing thinking. For these people, there are only yes and no answers, only right ways and wrong ways. This kind of thinking can make it difficult to solve problems, work in a team environment, collaborate, or even understand the perspective of another person. Adults who struggle with this kind of thinking can become oppositional and defiant when their opinion of "the right way" to do something is challenged. They are likely to avoid people who disagree with them and will have difficulty accepting changes that don't align with the way they view things.

This can result in confrontation, interpersonal relationship issues, and difficulty working in a team. It can also cause issues even when the person is performing work or making decisions on their own. They may decide that the only way to do the report their boss requested is to spend five days interviewing employees and conducting research, even though this is well beyond the scope and expectation of the boss's actual request.

All or nothing thinking can also lead to a kind of perfectionism that can be paralyzing and cause procrastination. In these circumstances, the person establishes their idea of "the perfect solution," and if that solution cannot be achieved, they will struggle to put any effort into the task at all since it either has to be all – the perfect solution – or nothing.

Memory Challenges

People with ADHD often struggle with several different kinds of memory. First, there is working memory. This is the kind of memory that you use throughout the day so that you can read a report and then take the information you learned and create a summary. Working memory and short-term memory are often used synonymously, although in some contexts they are slightly different. When ADHD adults have difficulties with working memory, it can lead to forgetfulness, decrease productivity, and make it challenging to figure out where they left their keys.

ADHD adults can also struggle with prospective memory, which is the type of memory that helps them remember to do things at some point in the future, like taking their workout clothes with them in the morning so they can go to the gym after work. Difficulties with prospective memory can also contribute to forgetfulness, missed appointments and deadlines, and failing to meet the expectations of those around them. Prospective memory challenges are also one of the reasons ADHD adults can struggle to learn from past mistakes.

ADHD adults can also struggle with long-term memory, primarily if they also struggle with inattention. The brain only stores those things that were deemed important enough to capture and sustain its attention. This means that adults with ADHD are unlikely to remember things they did not pay attention to.

Time Management

Many adults with ADHD have issues maintaining a sense of time. Time can pass more slowly or more quickly depending on what they are engaged in doing. Other factors, like struggling with planning and being forgetful, can make it challenging to get out of the house on time. Adults with ADHD who struggle with their sense of time will be consistently late for work, doctor's appointments, family activities, important events, and just about everything else.

This type of time management issue can also be seen in their inability to perform tasks in a timely fashion. Adults with ADHD may have difficulty meeting deadlines, paying bills on time, or accomplishing time-sensitive tasks like filing taxes.

What causes ADHD in Adults?

Based on the current available research, there is no clear answer to this question. Past studies indicate that there is a strong genetic component with ADHD, and that those with a first-degree relative with ADHD are five times more likely to have it as someone without a first-degree relative with the disorder. Other research indicates that mothers of ADHD children are 24 times more likely to have ADHD as mothers without ADHD children, and fathers with ADHD children are five times more likely than other fathers to have the condition.

Previously, research into the difference in dopamine levels between those with ADHD and those without the disorder seemed to point to this chemical imbalance as the root cause of the disorder. However, new research shows that the difference in dopamine levels is more likely to be another symptom than the actual cause of the disorder. It is most likely that ADHD is caused by a combination of factors that includes a genetic disposition.

While there are many other factors people believe may contribute to the development of ADHD, there isn't any scientific backing that any of the following cause ADHD in adults or children:

- Food dye
- Sugar
- Parenting
- Lead exposure
- Second-hand smoke
- Brain injury

How is Adult ADHD Diagnosed?

ADHD in adults must be diagnosed by a licensed mental health professional or a medical doctor. At this point, there is no medical or standardized testing that can definitively diagnose the disorder. Doctors and mental health professionals have a series of tools they can use to assist in the diagnosis process.

These tools are used to determine if the symptoms that can be documented are sufficient to meet the diagnostic criteria for adults according to the DSM-V which is outlined below:

1. Displays five or more of the symptoms outlined in either the list of inattentive symptoms or the list of hyperactive symptoms outlined below that have persisted for at least six months and are maladaptive to normal behavior.

Inattentive List

- Fails to pay attention to details, makes careless mistakes, overlooks details, or produces work that is inaccurate.
- Has difficulty sustaining attention while performing tasks, participating in conversations, or attending lectures or other events where attention is required.
- Seems not to be listening when spoken to directly, may appear to be tuned out or daydreaming.
- Fails to follow instructions and to follow-through and finish assigned work and household tasks.
- Struggles with organizing tasks and activities, sequencing tasks or events, and keeping belongings in order. Produces messy, unorganized work and struggles with tardiness, missed deadlines, and time management.

- Avoids starting tasks or activities that require sustained attention.
- Loses important items that are necessary for tasks or activities like cell phones, keys, wallets.
- Easily distracted by external stimuli.
- Forgets to perform daily activities like paying bills, returning calls, and running errands.

Hyperactive List

- Fidgets, taps hands or feet, struggles to sit still.
- Fails to remain seated when appropriate, like during meetings, at lectures.
- Feels restless.
- Struggles to participate in leisure activities quietly.
- Feels as if "driven by a motor."
- Talks excessively.
- Blurts out answers or statements, interrupts other people, struggles to wait for their turn to talk in a conversation.
- Has difficulty waiting in line or traffic.
- Interrupts other people's conversations and activities, uses other people's things without permission, or intrudes on others personal space.

2. Several of the inattentive or hyperactive-impulsive behaviors listed above must have been present prior to age 12.

3. Several inattentive or hyperactive-impulsive symptoms must be present in at least two settings – like at work and at home.

4. Clear evidence must be provided that the symptoms being experienced interfere with or reduce the quality

of the person's ability to function socially, academically, or occupationally.

5. The symptoms do not occur alongside schizophrenia or any other psychotic disorder and cannot be attributed to another mental health condition.

If a person meets all the diagnostic criteria, they can be diagnosed with ADHD, according to the guidelines provided by the DSM-V. When a diagnosis is made, the professional providing the diagnosis is required to categorize the severity of the person's ADHD as follows:

- Mild: The person has few symptoms beyond the minimum number required for a diagnosis and only experiences minor impairment because of these symptoms.
- Moderate: The person has more symptoms and experiences more impairment that someone that would be categorized as "mild," but does not meet the threshold to be considered "severe."
- Severe: The person has significantly more symptoms than is required for diagnosis and experiences significant impairment because of those symptoms.

One of the important things to note about the criteria is the requirement that symptoms were present prior to age 12. This highlights the fact that even if ADHD is diagnosed when someone is an adult, the disorder always begins in childhood. In fact, in order to get an ADHD diagnosis, symptoms have to have been present during childhood. For this reason, one of the first tools used in adult ADHD diagnosis is often a questionnaire that is used to determine if the symptoms were present in adolescence. The person handling the assessment may also ask for primary school report cards, information from parents, and a complete history of symptoms from the person being diagnosed.

Most diagnosticians will also inquire about the person's family history with ADHD because of the strong genetic component.

Although there are not definitive tests for ADHD, blood tests, neurological exams and scans, a series of psychological tests, and a complete medical exam may also be conducted in order to rule out other medical, neurological, and psychological problems.

Treating Adult ADHD

The Traditional Approach

The most common way that adult ADHD is treated by traditional medicine is with the use of medication. Research indicates that more than 60% of adults who take stimulant medication experience improvement in their symptoms. The kind of medication used to treat ADHD in adults is the same medication used to treat children including Adderall, Ritalin, Strattera, Concerta, Vyvanse, and Focalin.

However, medication is not effective for all people with ADHD. As many as 20% experience no symptom improvement at all with any medication used to treat the disorder. Additionally, anyone who has previously had a problem with substance abuse may be a bad candidate for stimulant medication. For these people, Strattera can be used because it can alleviate symptoms, but it is not a stimulant.

Even those who experience relief may opt not to take these medications due to the side effects which can vary widely from person to person.

While medication is often the first line of treatment, it is generally accepted that medication plus behavioral coaching and counseling can provide more benefit than either medication or behavioral programs alone.

The Alternative Options

Whether an individual chooses to use medication or not, there are several natural ways to treat ADHD and manage its symptoms. Some of the most common and effective natural treatments for ADHD are:

- ADHD Coaching - Life coaching to establish routines and develop strategies for managing symptoms
- Stress Management - Relaxation and stress management techniques like meditation, deep breathing, and massage
- Therapy - Individual cognitive behavioral therapy, group therapy, family therapy, and couples counseling
- Lifestyle Adjustments – Including sleep, diet, and exercise

While the use of stimulant medication is the most common course of treatment for adult ADHD, those wishing to follow a more natural and holistic path can use these alternative treatment options to manage symptoms and mitigate their effects on everyday life.

For a more detailed look at how to use natural treatment options to treat your ADHD, check out "***Managing ADHD: Take Control of ADHD Naturally***" from my ***Natural Health & Natural Cures Series.***

Conclusion

Thank you again for purchasing this book!

I hope it was valuable to you in providing a foundational understanding of adult ADHD.

The next step is to learn about how to manage the symptoms related to ADHD naturally and without the use of powerful stimulant medication. Understanding and knowledge are the best medicine!

Finally, if you enjoyed this book, please take the time to share your thoughts and post a review on Amazon. It'd be greatly appreciated!

Thank you and good luck!

Christine Weil

Check out some of Christine's other books!!!

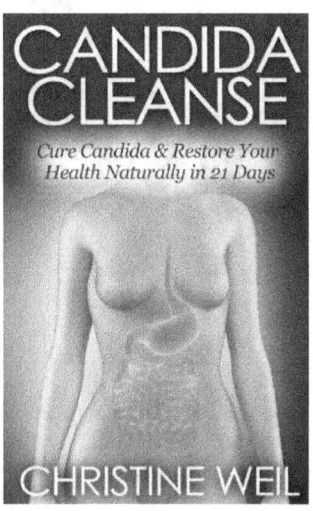

http://www.amazon.com/dp/B00IIRQH9K

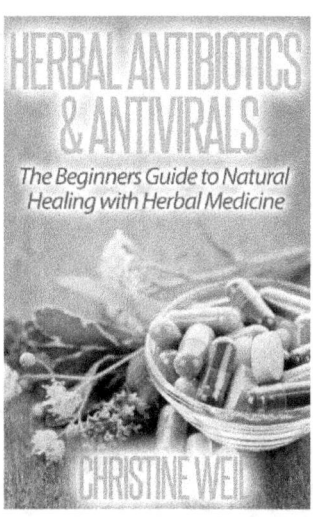

http://www.amazon.com/dp/B00J2F1QDO

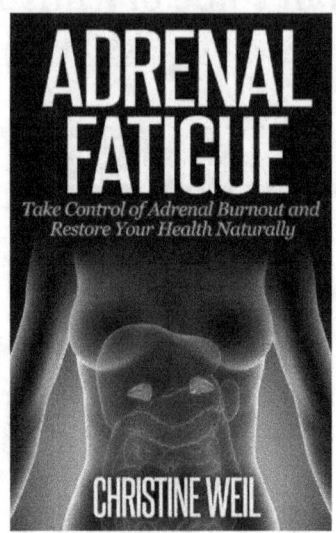

http://www.amazon.com/dp/B00J8SHS6E

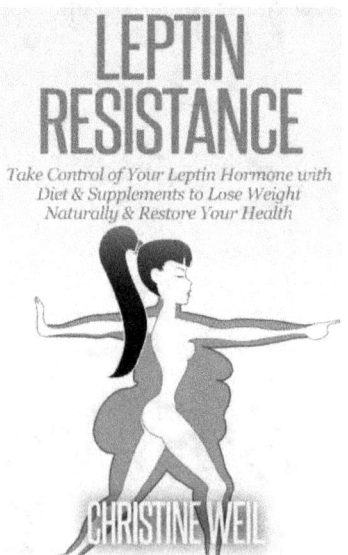

http://www.amazon.com/dp/B00J8UNBWW

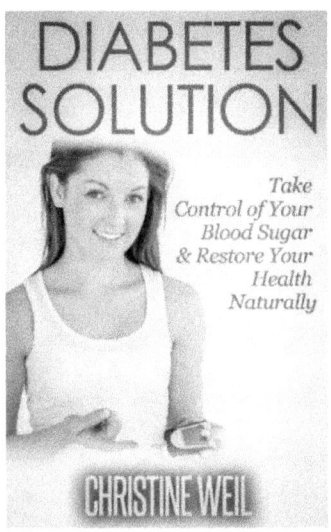

http://www.amazon.com/dp/B00KCAAKOO

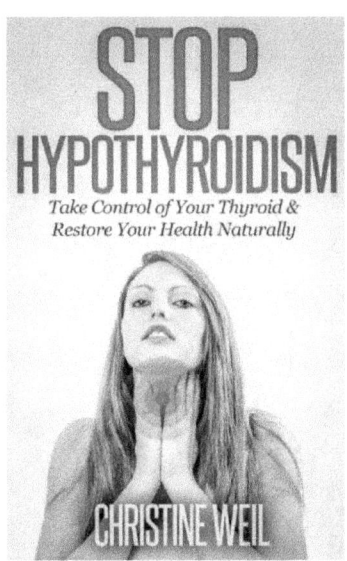

http://www.amazon.com/dp/B00KGI6TEC

www.ingramcontent.com/pod-product-compliance
Lightning Source LLC
Chambersburg PA
CBHW070514290526
45790CB00003B/1233